THE LITTLE BOOK OF

KINDNESS

Everyday actions to change your life and the world around you

BERNADETTE RUSSELL

First published in Great Britain in 2017 by Orion Spring
an imprint of The Orion Publishing Group Ltd
Carmelite House, 50 Victoria Embankment
London EC4Y 0DZ

An Hachette UK Company

1 3 5 7 9 10 8 6 4 2

The 'starfish story' retold by my friend Pete Sainsbury
on page 44 was inspired by Loren Eiseley's essay 'The Star Thrower',
published in 1969 in *The Unexpected Universe*.

A CIP catalogue record for this book is available from the British Library.

ISBN: 978 1 4091 7261 1

Printed in Great Britain by CPI Group (UK) Ltd, Croydon, CR0 4YY

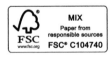

www.orionbooks.co.uk

CONTENTS

INTRODUCTION

*T*his book is about kindness. What it means, why it's important, and how it's good for you. It's also about how being kind can be fun, life-transforming; even world-changing.

I want to start by telling you how it all began for me. I was at the Edinburgh Festival in August 2011 with *Etherdome*, a comedy I had written about the development of anaesthetics in nineteenth-century America. (I know, it doesn't sound like much of a laugh, but trust me, it was hilarious.) On the morning of the 7th, I was in the City Cafe on Blair Street, eating breakfast and chatting with my friends about that day's plans. Behind us on a TV, the news was on. The images were shocking. We saw London in chaos: a double decker bus on fire, live footage of people kicking-in shop windows and looting, riot police, broken glass everywhere, groups of people running down the street smashing everything in their path, setting buildings on fire as they ran. The riots spread, from Tottenham to Brixton, Peckham, all places I knew and loved, and where my friends lived. Later they travelled, to Birmingham, Manchester, Bristol, and people locked themselves in their homes, full of fear, or else spilled out onto the streets, full of rage. It continued for five days. We couldn't take our eyes off it. We cried. We watched it endlessly, with our mouths wide open. We talked about what should be done, what could be done, why it was happening. We called home and checked in on people we knew and cared about.

Meanwhile, Mark Duggan, the young man who had been killed in Tottenham and whose death caused the protest at the beginning of these events, was mostly forgotten as commentators were asked to make sense of it all. Then things got even nastier. There were calls by a terrified public for water cannons to be utilised. There were journalists suggesting the rioters should be 'clubbed like baby seals', racist comments on chat shows, most of the blame for the disturbances piled onto the young and the poor.

However, there were many moments of light in this darkness. Monika Konczyk, a newcomer to London who was trapped and terrified at the top of her burning building, jumped and was safely caught and comforted. A fund was established for Maurice Reeves from Croydon, whose family's furniture shop was destroyed, to help them rebuild their premises. In nearby Peckham, thousands of sticky notes were stuck to a wall by local people, asking for peace, expressing love of their community, and an end to the destruction of the last few nights. On Twitter, Dan

Thompson started #riotcleanup, calling for people to help clear up the mess created by the riots, and hundreds of people armed with brooms and bags joined in. We watched all of this unfold too.

I came back to London from Edinburgh as planned, wondering what to expect. Everything looked the same. But nothing felt the same. I went to see Mr Patel, who runs the shop next door. He said his cousin's shop in Croydon had been ruined. I felt so sad for him and for everyone else. I kept thinking about the big mess we were in, from environmental troubles to wars and conflict and famines and endangered species and . . . the list went on and on. I wondered if there was any point to what I was doing; writing plays about Victorian-era dentists in a world with such troubles in it. I asked myself what I could do in the face of all this. On that day my answer was: nothing. There was literally nothing I could do that would make any difference. I'd be a fool to even try.

The next day, 18 August 2011, I was in the queue at our local post office. In front of me in the queue was a young man. He got to the counter and I overheard him say he'd forgotten his money, and that he'd been hoping to post his driving licence application. So, without thinking, I said, 'I'll pay for it.' It cost me a bit of loose change for a stamp, no big deal. He said, 'Thanks very much' and went on his way.

I thought about what had just happened. I thought maybe what I had done had cheered him up a bit. I realised it definitely had cheered me up, because I had very easily been able to make a tiny difference to another person. So when I got home I said to my partner, 'I've decided I know what to do.'

'About what?'

'About everything.'

'OK . . .'

'I'm going to do a kind thing for a stranger every day. For 366 days to cover the leap year. I'm going to see if kindness can change the world.'

And that was that. This fool tried! What followed was the most amazing, inspiring, joyous, life-affirming, terrifying, nerve-wracking, transformative and wonderful year of my life. To say it changed everything in my life would not be an exaggeration. During the year, I learned many valuable lessons which I will write about later in this book. But to sum up before we begin, believe me: being kind to yourself, to strangers, to those you love, to the world – every day, at every opportunity – will make you happier and more connected to everything and everyone than you have ever been. It will bring you peace, comfort and cake (I did receive a lot of cake, it's true).

We've always needed kindness . . .
But I believe right now . . . kindness is
more important than ever.

We've always needed kindness. But I believe right now, when we seem simultaneously more connected and more disconnected than ever before, when we are bombarded with negative images and messages about our fellow human beings, when we urgently need to listen to each other and find compromises where we disagree, when we all would like an end to war and to the damage of this planet, our home, when we need to imagine a brighter future and have faith in ourselves and each other, kindness is more important than ever.

Feel free to read this book in the order it is written, but it will work just as well if you dip in and out at any point. Do let me know what you have done and discovered – you can tweet me @betterussell, or with the hashtag #bekind.

But before you start, here are some examples of how kindness will change your life for the better:

Being kind makes you happy

Simply put, when you commit an act of kindness, it causes elevated levels of dopamine in the brain, which gives you a natural high: that's what that fuzzy warm feeling is. You can try this experiment on yourself, and notice how being kind makes you feel. You feel good partly because you can say to yourself, 'I did that, that's who I am, a kind person', and be proud of that. You will find you think better of yourself and others, because you will start to notice kindness all around you. You will become more positive about human beings in general, and you will feel empowered. Your life will most probably become more interesting. Plus, you will have fun.

Doing something out of the goodness of your heart, protects your heart

Really. It does. Being kind produces the hormone oxytocin in the brain and throughout the body. Oxytocin releases nitric oxide in blood vessels, which expands the blood vessels. This reduces blood pressure, thereby protecting your heart.

Kindness keeps you young

Research has shown that oxytocin, produced by the fuzzy warm feelings we have when we are kind, reduces levels of free radicals and inflammation in the cardiovascular system. These two are the main culprits that speed up the ageing process, and being kind combats them. It's kind people who are truly young at heart (and everywhere else).

Kindness helps all human beings

When you are kind to someone, you feel a connection with them, and you create a bond. Our ancestors had to learn to co-operate with each other to survive, and a group with very strong bonds had a much greater chance of survival. That's as true now as it was thousands of years ago. We human beings have kindness in our genes.

Kindness is contagious

When we're kind, we inspire others to be kind. My experience is proof of this – every day since I started, someone, somewhere will contact me with a story of a kindness they have committed or received. So be kind, share your stories and watch how you inspire others.

Make a start now. Have fun x

Bernadette Russell

CHAPTER 1

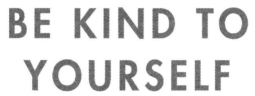

BE KIND TO YOURSELF

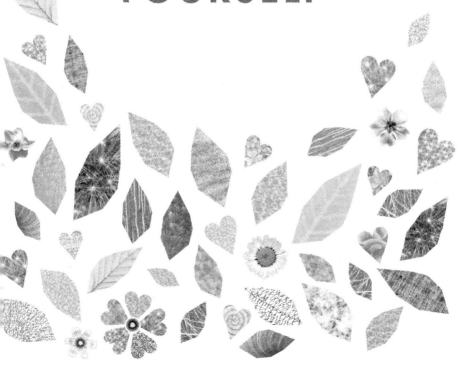

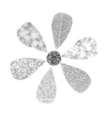

Being kind to yourself isn't always as easy as it sounds. Most of us are incredibly hard on ourselves. Pay attention to the kinds of thoughts you have about yourself in the course of an ordinary day. You miss the train and your inner critic pipes up with, 'You idiot, why didn't you leave the house earlier?' You're getting ready in the morning and you say to yourself, 'You look so fat/gaunt/ugly/weird.' Even when you're with friends and family you might be thinking, 'He/she doesn't really like me, I'm so boring.' If you had a friend who spoke to you like that, you'd be wise to start keeping your distance.

You may be one of those people who already speak to yourself gently and with compassion. If so: great, keep it up. But if, like most of us, you are your own worst critic, you need to make a conscious effort to stop; first by noticing, and then by changing it. Try talking to yourself with this in mind, out loud if you're able to find a space. If you've had a bad day, try: 'That is awful, sorry that happened. Tomorrow will be better, you deserve it to be.' Give yourself a hug (I know, this sounds daft. Try it). Recognise that what you are experiencing is normal, you are not alone, and that life is challenging sometimes. Notice and accept both positive and negative emotions; they're both part of being human.

366 days

Being kind to myself was an important lesson for me to learn. Halfway through my first year of daily acts of kindness, after having walked for forty minutes in flip-flops to help a woman struggling to get her very heavy shopping home (I'd just popped out for a pint of milk, hence the flimsy footwear) I felt weary, defeated, and convinced my arms had stretched to the length of a gibbon's. I didn't want to burn out, so I decided to try to be a little bit kinder on myself, enabling me to continue my mission. I had a swim, and then went on a day trip to Brighton to meet an old friend.

This chapter sets out a few practical exercises to help you on your way to being kind to yourself, all tried and tested by me. As my wise friend told me at the end of a difficult day, 'Your unhappiness will not improve the world, so if you can, be happy.' If you are kind to yourself at every opportunity, I am sure that you will be happier. Then you'll be ready to spread kindness into the wider world.

HAPPY BOOK

Get yourself a small notebook; this will be your 'Happy Book'. Find a quiet space and ten minutes' alone time. Write down everything that makes you happy, no matter how small. For example: walking the dog, watching the rain on the window from inside, lying in on Sunday . . .

Add to your 'Happy Book' as often as you can. If a week has passed and you haven't done at least one thing from the book every day, then you aren't being kind enough to yourself. If you've no money then find the things on the list that are free (e.g. dancing). If you've no time, find the things on the list that don't eat up valuable hours (e.g. listening to music on the way to work). Assuming, of course, that the things you've chosen are legal, not injurious to your or anybody else's health and don't include the phrase 'space travel', as this might not be realistic, use your list every day.

MIRROR MIRROR ON THE WALL . . .

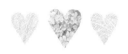

Many of us measure our self-worth by how we look. The morning scrutiny in the mirror is a great opportunity to combat the self-critic and start being kinder to yourself. When you can be sure of some alone time, look at yourself in the mirror. Now list ten things that you love about yourself, without conditions ('I like the colour of my eyes', 'I have a lovely smile', 'I am strong', etc.). Take as long as it takes. Write them down, if that helps, or just remember them if you're good at that. Then, aloud (again, I know it may seem silly, but you deserve it, trust me) speak to yourself in the mirror and tell yourself all of those ten things. If you absolutely can't make it to ten then you must ask your nearest and dearest to add to your list, but you should try to get there yourself if you can. I'd recommend doing this whenever your physical confidence is at a low. By the way, none of us is perfect. The good news is — we don't need to be.

THE WINNER IS . . .

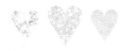

You may sometimes find yourself thinking, 'I'm not good/ clever/witty/educated/fit enough.' Some of these self-criticisms may be true, but part of being kind to yourself is celebrating what you *are* good at. Doing this will improve your confidence, and then you'll be ready to work on the areas you feel you need and would like to.

Write a list of your own achievements and skills. Imagine an awards ceremony for life; what might you win an award for? On this auspicious occasion you have actually won in ten categories, all of them focused on your personal talents and skills. These categories can be anything you excel at, from making people laugh, to always remembering birthdays, to being able to swim a mile, etc. If you are stuck, ask friends and family to help. Write them down, and keep the list in your wallet or purse. Sneak a peek when you need to remember what you are good at. Add to the list when you think of more, or when someone praises you for something.

START YOUR LIST OF ACHIEVEMENTS HERE:

QUICK-FIRE EXERCISES TO TRY

Laugh – hang out with funny people, watch funny films, read funny books, go and see some live comedy. Laugh until you have tummy ache. Be silly.

Get moving – work out at the gym, go for a walk, swim, or dance to your favourite song in the kitchen.

Eat – healthy eating is a way of being kind to yourself. Treating yourself now and then is also a kindness. 'A little of what you fancy does you good', as the old saying goes.

Treat – ask yourself what you're missing. If it's time alone, then make it happen; if it's sleep, ask someone to help you with the morning chores so you can lie in. Check your Happy Book (page 14) and treat yourself.

Inspiration – spend a bit of time at the beginning and end of each day seeking out something uplifting. Find the good news.

Say no – if yes comes easily and your life is wearisome because of it.

Say yes – if no comes easily and you wish your life were more exciting.

Know that if you are kind to yourself you will be happier, and that your happiness in itself is a gift to the world.

You will notice that
happiness, like kindness,
is contagious.

CHAPTER 2

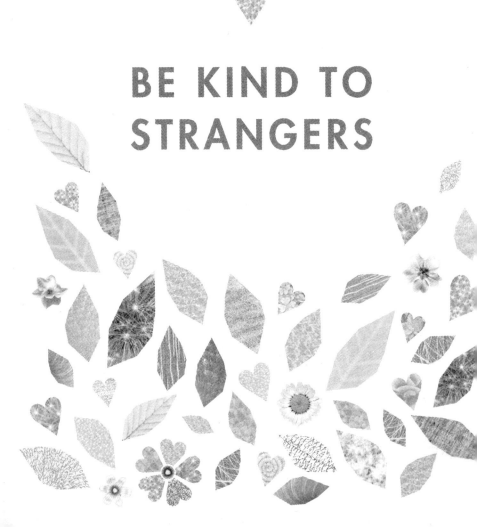

BE KIND TO STRANGERS

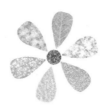

*I*n the distant past, when we lived in small hunter-gatherer communities, strangers were treated with suspicion and we were kind to our tightly knit group exclusively. It was tough out there; we had to help each other to survive.

Things are very different now. Few of us live with small groups of people whom we have known all our lives, on whom we are dependent for everything. Nowadays, we rarely know our neighbours, and seldom stay in the town

Being kind to strangers can make you more connected to the world you live in: challenge your preconceptions, and take your mind off your own troubles.

we grew up in. Most of us live in urban environments with transitory communities, which can be lonely and isolating.

To perform a kindness for a stranger who most probably won't see you again, when you have no possibility of being rewarded for that kindness, is an act that has the power to change someone's life.

You can't know what effect your kindness might have, but you can be sure that in a small way you have improved someone's life, even if it's just by giving a seat to a weary commuter.

If you would like to live in a kinder, happier, more peaceful world, the good news is you can help make that happen, simply by doing and being those things yourself.

366 days

About halfway through my year of kindness I was having serious doubts about whether what I was doing was actually doing any good. Because my daily acts of kindness were for strangers, I never heard anything back. Around this time I asked if anyone wanted to nominate someone who needed cheering up, and my friend Denise suggested sending something to her friend Stewart, who had been feeling very low since a recent hip operation. I sent him a homemade card with an encouraging message inside. Months passed. Denise told me Stewart had got the card and had loved it. I got in touch and asked if we could meet, and we did a few weeks later. He told me: 'You don't need much to feel better when you feel super-low. All you need is a smile or a kind word; the ripple effect that it has is enormous.' He said that receiving the card marked the beginning of him feeling less depressed, that soon after he started to get out and about a bit more. I benefited from meeting Stewart so much too: it gave me the confidence to continue my mission in the knowledge that a small act of kindness to a stranger can have a very positive effect.

SPREAD THE LOVE

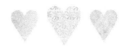

On Valentine's Day 2012, some friends and I delivered 150 homemade Valentine's cards to total strangers all around London. Our mission was to reclaim Valentine's Day as a festival of love for humanity. Most people loved it. A couple of people ran away, probably thinking we were selling something or trying to get them to sign something. One man swore at me. But we were also showered with hugs, smiles, free coffee, free wine and many, many thanks. Throughout the day we experienced joy, elation and exhaustion, as we travelled from Deptford to the bars of Soho, to Holloway Prison and Hampstead Heath. We met a milkman, several police officers, a man dressed in a foam mobile-phone costume doing promotions in the rain, couples and families, tourists and office workers, builders and homeless people, even an opera singer dressed in a gold velvet coat. We met many strangers and we put a smile on many faces. Every year since then I've revived this tradition, and it is a great reminder that most people are friendly, nice and open. There are some, of course, who don't want a free homemade card with a jelly heart stuck on top, and that's fair enough. As much as I would love you to do something similar next Valentine's Day, there are many less strenuous and equally rewarding ways of being kind to strangers. You don't have to go out of your comfort zone or be an extrovert. Go easy on yourself to begin with.

Start by simply trying to think the best of people. Focus on what we all have in common as human beings. We all need to eat and sleep; we all need shelter and love. We all have bad days. It's not nice when the man at the train station pushes past you, but it is worth reminding yourself that you have no idea what he is going through. Notice when people are suffering.

Start by simply trying
to think the best of people.

Before you begin

When approaching strangers, try saying something like:
'Hello, I'm trying to do a good deed whenever I can;
I wondered if you'd help me out?' (Almost everyone gets
the concept of a 'good deed'.)

Start to notice when you can help strangers out and take the opportunity to do so. A great start is on your daily journey to and from work or school.

Smile

We can all treat strangers the way we would like to be treated ourselves, and make our little patch of the world kinder. Try this for starters: smile and say good morning to everyone you see. Do this every day for a week to begin with, and make a note of how many smiles you gave out each day, how many you got back, and how you felt in response to that. For fun, try to beat your previous day's record or the number of reciprocated smiles. Some of these smiles might turn into conversations and some of the people you smile at you may start to notice every day; they might even become friends.

A helping hand

There are loads of things you can do to make a stranger's day that little bit easier. Keep an eye out for opportunities to be kind. Spend one week experimenting with being kind at every opportunity on your daily journeys. Keep a diary of what you did and when, what sort of reactions you got and how it made you feel. Try: offering to help carry heavy luggage, bags or buggies; holding a door open for someone; offering someone your seat; noticing if someone looks lost and helping with directions; passing on a newspaper or magazine when you've finished reading it; holding the lift for someone; letting someone have your parking space; letting someone in front of you in the queue for the bus or train.

KINDNESS CHECK-OUT

Now you've had some practice, try these when you're in less of a rush to get somewhere – make a note of what you did, where, and what kind of reaction you got. Tick these off as you do them and enjoy seeing how many you have tried out.

○ Ask the person at the check-out how they are – have a chat

○ Tell your delivery person they are doing a great job

○ Leave some credit in the vending machine for the next person

○ Leave a note of thanks to your server (plus a tip!)

○ Help someone struggling to reach stuff on the top shelf in the supermarket

○ If you notice someone in distress, ask if they're OK or need help

○ Offer your change to someone struggling to find the right amount

○ Tell visitors all the best things to do and see in your area

KINDNESS IS MAGIC

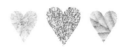

OK, so now you've had some practice and are feeling more confident, have a go at these cheeky missions – you'll probably have some ideas of your own, too. Again, keep a note of what you did, where you did it, and how it made you feel.

○ When you buy a coffee, pay for two so the next person gets theirs for free

○ Leave a friendly note inside a book at the library

○ Leave a note under a windscreen wiper saying, 'I hope you have a nice day'

○ Leave kind notes in public places, such as on bathroom mirrors, with messages like, 'You are loved'

○ Write a friendly letter to a stranger and leave it in a public place with '*Please read me*' on the envelope

○ Deliver Christmas/holiday/New Year cards to strangers

○ Give away an umbrella on a rainy day

○ Give a stranger a lottery ticket

BE A KINDNESS SUPERHERO

Try these out, and think about what superpowers you'd choose if you could change the world for the better.

- Talk to the person at the party who is on their own – you never know what an incredible, life-changing conversation you may have with them.
- Stick up for someone if they are being bullied/harassed.
- Be ever vigilant for who might need help or your kindness!

Notice the kindness of strangers

Spend a whole day noting every time a stranger is kind to you. Pay attention to strangers being kind to each other and enjoy observing this.

QUICK-FIRE ROUND

- Pay someone a compliment. (Nerve-wracking, but I have literally never known this not to put a smile on someone's face. It's good to focus on those who might not get compliments so often.)
- Talk to strangers. Good icebreakers are weather and sport.
- Try a 'hello, how are you?' to the next stranger you see.

The smallest act of kindness
is worth more than
the grandest intention.

OSCAR WILDE

CHAPTER 3

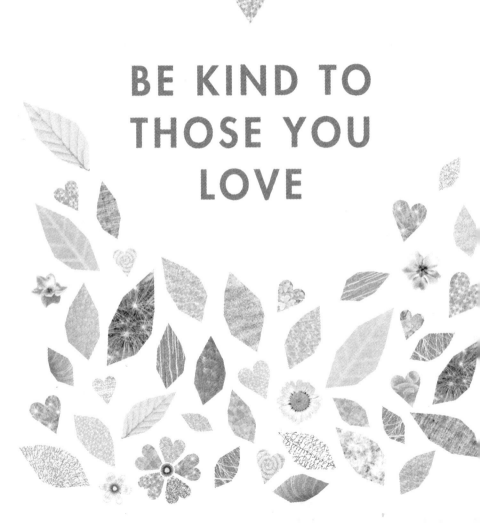

BE KIND TO THOSE YOU LOVE

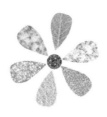

*B*eing kind to our friends and family is something we expect to be a minimum requirement of a decent human being. In fact, it is incredibly easy to take the people closest to us for granted, and to be unintentionally neglectful and unkind. We're all so busy that it can take months to arrange to meet an old friend for a coffee, weeks can fly by and you realise that you haven't spoken to your best friend or to your parents, and we sometimes hardly have enough time for those we live with.

We can choose to redefine a successful life by how much we've learned, how much joy we've experiences, how much happiness we have brought to others.

Our definition of success (a bigger salary, a more important-sounding job title, fancier possessions, etc.) has resulted in us working longer hours, sleeping with our phones within arm's reach and missing important moments with those closest to us. We all have to pay the rent and put food on the table, and that can be a struggle sometimes, but we can choose to redefine a successful life by how much we've learned, how much joy we've experienced, how much happiness we have brought to others and what we have done to make the world a better place.

LEARN TO LISTEN

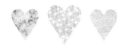

One of the best ways of being kind to your loved ones is by active, compassionate listening. We can all be guilty of not really listening but simply hearing, just by waiting for the other person to stop speaking so it is our turn.

Try this: next time you ask someone how they are, listen and don't interrupt. Try to resist giving advice unless it's asked for: ask questions instead. Give the person as much time as they need.

My friend Richard was telling me all about how he was considering giving in his notice at work. He told me work had become so stressful that he had insomnia, felt constantly anxious and was totally unappreciated by his boss. I was listening, but I was also thinking about how I could make him feel better by sharing an example of a similar experience that I'd had. Then he said, 'I don't want a solution. I just want to moan for five minutes.' I'm so glad he told me that; it was a bit of a turning point for me.

Now I work on actively listening, especially with friends and family. People don't always need your advice; instead it may be a shoulder to cry on or for you to say 'well done'. It's worth remembering that some people talk a lot because they don't feel listened to enough, or because they're lonely, or because they need to work something out aloud. Give them time to talk. Whether it's hearing their problems or just news of their day, pay attention and listen.

366 days

My friend had had a very bad week. We all have those weeks sometimes. We'd spoken on the phone but both had very busy schedules and didn't manage to meet up. I wanted to do something to cheer her up. I had a copy of her house keys, so I snuck in whilst she was out, and left flowers, a bottle of wine and a 'welcome home' note on the table for when she got in, like a benevolent burglar. It was really good fun, and she absolutely loved it.

KINDNESS TOP TEN

Make home the best place to be by trying these simple acts of kindness for those you love – tick them off when you have done each one and make a note of the reaction you got. Ask them to score each out of ten and you'll know what works best!

○ Treat them to breakfast in bed

○ Do a chore that they normally do so they don't have to do it

○ Make them their favourite dinner (and pudding)

○ Make your home beautiful for them for when they get back

○ Make them a playlist of music they'll like

○ Clean their room as a surprise

○ Leave them notes in their lunch box, in the fridge, on their pillow, in the bathroom, to make them smile

○ When they've been away, make them a 'welcome home' banner

○ Be on time and say sorry if you're not

○ Throw a surprise dinner party with their favourite people

SAY IT,
DON'T JUST THINK IT

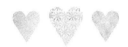

At the very next opportunity, take time to tell your loved one all the many things they are good at, and all the many things which make them so special to you. Too often we think these things but don't say them, sometimes taking it for granted that people will just know. Then write this down, in a good old-fashioned love letter (this doesn't have to be for your significant other; you can write a loving letter to a friend or relative too). Have a think about how they would most enjoy receiving it — you could hand deliver it, stick it in the post, or leave it somewhere for them to discover it. It will always be something for them to look at, to remind them that they are loved and of all the things that make them special.

MAKE A DATE

Create an opportunity to have some time with your loved one to tell them about your life and ask them about their life, how they're feeling and what they need to be happy. Ask their opinion about things so they will know you value their thoughts. If they're having a bad time, listen. If they're having a great time, help them celebrate. Tell them they are loved; say sorry if you've done wrong. Remember it's also kind to tell people when they're behaving badly/drinking too much/making bad choices, but these things are better discussed with time and care than blurted out in frustration, so making time will help you to air any grievances or concerns. The most important thing is to make a date, and spend time in each other's company. You could get creative and make them an invitation. Aim to spend at least one day a month with someone you love having a proper catch-up.

The Story of Us

Write or draw in a scrapbook as a gift with photos and memories of the times you have spent together. You could prepare this as a birthday or holiday present, or as a gift for the anniversary of when you first met.

Big Day

Give them an extra special day: arrange a surprise day out for them and take them somewhere you know they have never been/to do something they've never done. Try reading them a story in bed (this works for any age!), giving them a massage, pouring them a bubble bath (and maybe a glass of wine). Create a new anniversary just for the two of you – 'best friend day', 'sisters' day', 'Auntie day' – whatever. A day for just you two to celebrate your relationship.

Surprise

Decorate the outside of their home with paper bunting, flowers and a homemade sign with their name and a kind message; redecorate a room for them or tidy up their garden; throw a surprise party for their birthday, homecoming or new job; give them a handmade gift; draw a picture; bake a cake; write a haiku; sing them 'Happy Birthday' in person or on the phone.

Kindness Call

Call someone you haven't spoken to for a while, just to let them know they mean a lot to you. Try to regularly call loved ones who live at a distance. Phone for no reason other than a chat. Try phoning someone who you think might be isolated or bored. Find out what the best time to call your loved ones is and make a note of it.

QUICK-FIRE ROUND

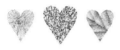

- Buy someone an unexpected gift.

- Babysit and give someone a night off.

- Pay attention to your loved ones' appearance and achievements — tell them they are beautiful or have done well.

- If you can spare it, give cash to someone who is struggling; tell them to pay you back whenever they are able with no pressure. Let them know you've been in the same boat so they don't feel bad.

- Encourage dreaming — assist your loved ones to pursue their hearts' desire, either practically (with job and college applications) or by cheering them on.

- Offer to spring-clean their home.

CHAPTER 4

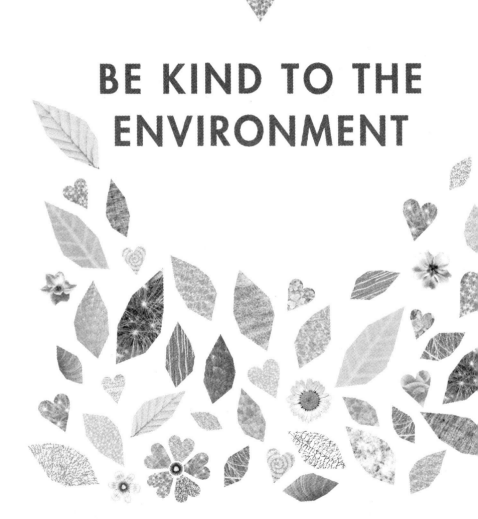

BE KIND TO THE ENVIRONMENT

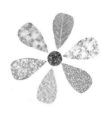

*R*eports of pollution, extinction and climate change can be pretty disheartening. There need to be major shifts in thinking at a governmental and corporate level on environmental issues, and we can help by signing petitions, joining campaigns, lobbying politicians, etc. But we can make changes too. Becoming more environmentally aware is one of the best ways we have of being kind to ourselves, each other, future generations and the other creatures we share the planet with.

Becoming more environmentally
aware is one of the best ways
we have of being kind.

366 days

My friend Pete told me a story (originally attributed to Loren Eiseley), to encourage me to continue my kindness mission. He said this best explained what kindness meant to him:

One day there was a little girl walking along the beach. The beach was filled with starfish, washed up on the sand. A man was walking on the beach too. He noticed that every so often she picked up a starfish and threw it into the water. When the man crossed paths with the little girl he said to her: 'There are thousands of starfish on this beach. It's nice, what you are doing, but it won't make any difference.' The little girl looked at the man, picked up a starfish, threw it into the water and said: 'Well, it made a difference to that one.'

I love this story because it reminds me that every act of kindness is significant. Sometimes the man in that story was the voice in my head asking 'what is the point?', and it served as a reminder to be more like the strong little girl, who does it anyway.

So here are some ideas, big and small, of how to be kind to the environment.

MINDFUL SHOPPING

Our love of buying new stuff uses loads of material resources and precious energy. It also creates pollution when those items are shipped around the world. We can be kind whilst we shop by choosing Fairtrade products and companies who are more transparent about their employment and environmental policies, which also helps to ensure people are paid fairly for their labour. Also check for the recycled logo on items you purchase – many products are clearly marked so you can choose those that are widely recycled and avoid those that aren't so easily.

- Experiment by buying nothing apart from the absolute essentials for a month. Notice the differences in your mood, your finances and your time.

- Reduce your carbon footprint by buying second-hand or 'pre-loved' items.

- Use charity shops, markets and online market sites.

- Switch from buying cheap/disposable stuff to quality items that will last, when you can afford to. Less landfill, fewer resources used in making stuff, and you'll save money in the long run. As the saying goes, 'buy cheap, buy twice'.

- Make do and mend – repair that broken toaster if you are able to.

- Be a borrower – no need to buy something, especially if you're only going to use it occasionally. Offer to lend and share your things too.

- When you *have* to replace items, look for energy-efficient appliances.

- Use rechargeable batteries. Disposables take up landfill space, plus they leak acid into the earth.

- Say no to plastic cutlery and other disposables – they use precious resources and spend centuries in landfills. Bring your own and reuse them.

- No aerosols – they're toxic to the environment and you. Buy pump sprays or creams.

- Have a clear-out – your old belongings will be welcome somewhere. Donate to charity shops, friends and neighbours. Sell them online or at a market – anything is better than taking them to the tip.

SHOP LESS: USE YOUR MONEY TO *DO* STUFF, NOT *HAVE* STUFF

Try this experiment for a month (tough for shopaholics, I know, but it's only one month!). Every time you are tempted by a new pair of shoes, gadget, game, etc.: don't buy it. Make a note of how much it would have cost you and put that money away somewhere, as if you had spent it. At the end of the month, tot up how much you would have spent, and use the money to do something you enjoy instead. Make a note of what you would have bought, how much you would have spent on the item, how much you 'saved' during the month and what you did with the money instead. (If you did this for a year, imagine what adventures you could have! And what could you do if you did this for a lifetime . . . ?)

SAVE WATER

There are more and more humans on the planet, but the same amount of drinkable water, so we have to be careful with it.

- Turn off the tap whilst cleaning your teeth.
- Collect rainwater in a waterproof container. Use it for watering plants.
- Only switch on a FULL washing machine/dishwasher.

Take showers, not baths. Sing your favourite three-minute pop song; then you'll know you're clean enough. Try a different 'shower song' every day for a week.

FOOD FOR THOUGHT

We waste *so* much food – enough globally to feed the one billion hungry people in the world. It ends up in landfills, turns into destructive methane, and is a waste of the water and energy that went into producing it.

Meat and dairy production is highly resource-intensive and inefficient – it uses a huge amount of water and energy and creates harmful greenhouse gas emissions too.

Give up meat and/or dairy for one day a week – one of the best things you can do for the environment and for your health. Check out the #MeatFreeMonday campaign started by Paul McCartney and his family; there's a website too, with recipes and ideas. Start a recipe collection of meals you've tried and enjoyed.

Also try these:

- Visit farmers' markets – buy local vegetables and fruits.

- Get local food delivered – buying food that is sourced locally reduces fuel use and therefore reduces pollution.

- Plan your meals for the week, so there's less chance of you wasting food or money.

- Get into leftover meals (usually the yummiest).

- If you eat out, take a container for what's left over to be packed up. Saves it being thrown away, and you'll have dinner for tomorrow!

- Grow your own – no fuel will be used in transportation, and you'll save money. Start with some herbs on a windowsill. Maybe you could consider getting an allotment – check out what is available locally.

SAVING ENERGY

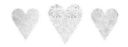

Most of the energy we depend on at present is finite and produces pollution – so we need to save it.

Walk

If you're able, use stairs, not lifts/escalators. Walk to local amenities. Start keeping a note of how far you have walked every day. At the end of the week/month/year calculate the distance – it's estimated that the average is around two miles a day, so try to beat it and achieve the recommended 10,000 steps (five miles). You could invest in a pedometer, or use an app on your phone to keep track of how you're doing.

Pick public transport

Buses, trains, trams, etc. are better for the environment (and a chance to chat to a stranger!).

Cycle

Biking instead of driving can reduce more than 90 per cent of greenhouse gas emissions. There are plenty of classes around to brush up your cycling skills.

Carpool

Reduce carbon emissions whilst getting to know your fellow travellers.

Fly less

Aeroplanes emit huge quantities of pollution. Consider going on holiday closer to home – you could try a walking or cycling holiday.

Switch over

Change from regular bulbs to energy-saving ones – they last longer and use only a quarter of the energy. Start with the lights you leave on the most.

Switch off

If you're not using it, turn it off. This includes lights, televisions, computers, printers, etc.

PLASTIC FANTASTIC

Plastic debris can injure and harm wildlife, particularly when ingested by marine animals. It releases toxic chemicals into the soil, and is not easily recycled.

- Buy reusable glass/metal water bottles and fill up from the tap. Remember, most tap water in developed countries is safe to drink.

- Use reusable shopping bags; carry a few with you ready for when you need them.

- Avoid plastic packaging – buy fruit and veggies from markets. Most people will be happy to put the goods straight into your bag. Avoid food that's individually wrapped. Buy in bulk – a huge bag of rice uses less plastic than ten small bags of rice.

- Take your own mug. We get through an estimated 2.5 billion disposable cups a year in the UK alone, so it could make a massive difference if we just carried our own travel cups. Some coffee shops even provide discounts for bringing your own mug.

GO WILD
QUICK-FIRE ROUND

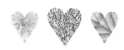

- 'Re-wild' your garden – use organic garden treatments and plant wildflowers.

- Create a compost – less food waste in landfills and richer soil for your garden.

- Plant your garden with bee-friendly flowers like lavender, snapdragons and hollyhocks.

- Volunteer at your local wildlife conservation group.

- Explore the woods, the parks, and the coast near where you live. Leave it as you found it and enjoy.

- Feed the birds – all year round. Check out the advice on the RSPB website for what grub is best for our feathered friends.

CHAPTER 5

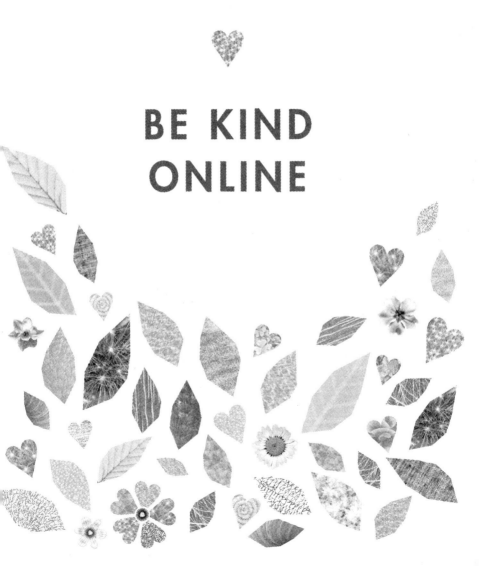

BE KIND
ONLINE

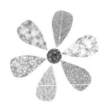

*T*he internet provides us with access to an incredible amount of information and knowledge, allowing us to reconnect with long-lost friends and enjoy a lot of cute animal videos, amongst many other things. It's possible to learn to do pretty much anything online, and to get advice and feedback on a seemingly infinite range of topics.

However, online debate can get heated pretty quickly. I began to notice a gap between how people discuss things online (quick to anger and judge each other, sometimes aggressive and rude) and how discussions happen in real life (often more calmly, good-humoured and generously). It seems that we still have a way to go in learning how to use the internet well and wisely.

But there is enormous potential for good online, massive scope for kindness towards others, and ourselves, with great opportunities for positive action that many individuals, groups and organisations have already tapped into. It's up to each of us to help make this work.

I used social media as a way of keeping a diary of my acts of kindness in my first year, learned about other people's ideas of kindness, and discovered fun ways of being kind online.

There is enormous potential for good online.

366 days

My friend Kirsty read on Facebook that I was trying out acts of kindness for strangers. Kirsty told me about her nana's best friend, who had felt lonely and isolated when Kirsty's nana had passed away. Kirsty gave me her address and I sent her a present. She said it cheered her up so much that a stranger could be so kind. Kirsty said this led to her nana's friend eventually having more confidence to go out of the house again and connect with people. This is just one very small example of something positive that social media helped happen.

ENJOY YOUR LIFE

Most people don't post pictures on Instagram of burnt Sunday roasts, or tweet about an average day at work when nothing much happened, or post a live video of them stubbing their toe whilst hunting for the TV remote on a Saturday night. Instead, we see selfies of beautiful happy faces, enviable views of paradise holidays and announcements of pregnancies, engagements and promotions. You could easily come to the conclusion that everyone has a better life than you. If this is making you feel down, then unfollow or mute those people who, intentionally or not, are making you feel bad. Stop torturing yourself. Meet up with a friend who makes you feel better, stronger and happier. Don't believe the hype.

CHANGE FOR GOOD

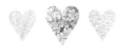

You might easily come to the conclusion that the world is a terrible place and humankind is doomed, as you scroll endlessly through news articles that look like trailers for the latest Armageddon-themed Hollywood blockbuster. Of course there is bad stuff in the world. It is important and useful to stay informed about current affairs, and do what we can to improve things. But there's also plenty of good stuff in the world, and it's worth remembering that there have ALWAYS been struggles, challenges and battles to fight. If you find that the news is draining all joy from your life, maybe it is time for a change.

Start by seeking out and sharing online positive stories that inspire you (they are out there). Good news doesn't have to be pictures of cats and foxes becoming best friends, although I'm a big fan of those too. Stories about humans being kind and doing good make us feel hopeful. So be kind by sharing these stories, and become a defender of hope.

USE IT
FOR THE POSITIVE

The internet can provide us with fantastic platforms for positive action: for simply sharing things we like; good news and useful information; and it can also be used for campaigning, petitions, organising events and fundraising. Use it to share things that are useful, helpful, truthful and kind.

Try this: for one week seek out things online that made you smile or feel more positive – these can be silly or serious, whatever appeals to you. Make a note on the next page of the stories you read and begin to change what you focus on. If this helps you, then commit to making it a daily practice, even if it is just one positive story a day.

10 QUICK-FIRE WAYS TO BE KIND ONLINE

1. Practise good 'netiquette'

Don't type in capital letters, as it's a bit LIKE BEING SHOUTED AT (see?). Be as nice as you would when interacting with someone face to face. Before you type, ask yourself: 'Is it true? Is it helpful? Is it necessary? Is it kind?' (P.S. The answers should all be yes).

2. Send short, polite emails

Many of us are overwhelmed by email spam, offers, invites and requests to send perfect strangers our bank details for a variety of dubious reasons. Keep it brief if you can. Don't get cross if you don't get immediate replies – there could be a very good reason for it.

3. Post good reviews

If you've bought something, visited a restaurant or been on holiday and loved it: share that experience and make it personal. If you haven't had a positive experience, where possible make direct contact with the organisation and let them know. They may not be aware of their shortcomings and it's probably useful for them to receive constructive criticism. Be gentle. Same goes for books, plays, exhibitions, films, etc. – leave the artists feedback if you've enjoyed their work.

4. Share good news

Share positive news stories every time you see or hear about them. Look for articles that highlight solutions rather than simply present problems. You might be sharing just the thing someone needed to cheer them up.

5. Think the best of people

Resist responding online with anger or criticism – sometimes the nicest people can come across as unreasonable. If you need to, move the discussion into the real world. Everybody has bad days.

6. Post funny stuff

Post funny videos. Be silly. Share jokes. Making someone laugh on- or offline is one of the best ways to be kind.

7. Practise positivity

Share other people's good news and help them celebrate. If you like a post, 'like' it! If you can think of something that will help – say it! Say congratulations, well done, Happy New Year, etc.

8. Fundraising

Support people who are fundraising by helping them spread the word. Start a campaign online yourself. A wonderful example recently ensured that a lady living in sheltered housing received some birthday cards – lots of people shared the post and she received hundreds from well-wishers. Use the internet as a global village noticeboard for good causes.

9. Share useful and positive information

Share your top tips: recipes, new places you've discovered, great bars, books, films, TV series, new shops and markets. Use social media to provide a platform for people to share news, ask for help and announce parties – a Facebook group, Twitter account, blog or website.

10. Follow online groups and communities who promote kindness

There are plenty more popping up every day. Have fun researching them.

There are lots of people who feel disconnected because they don't have access to, or feel confident in, using the internet. A great act of kindness is helping someone use this incredible resource by sharing your skill and knowledge. Lots of local libraries are keen to have volunteers who can help people skill up.

CHAPTER 6

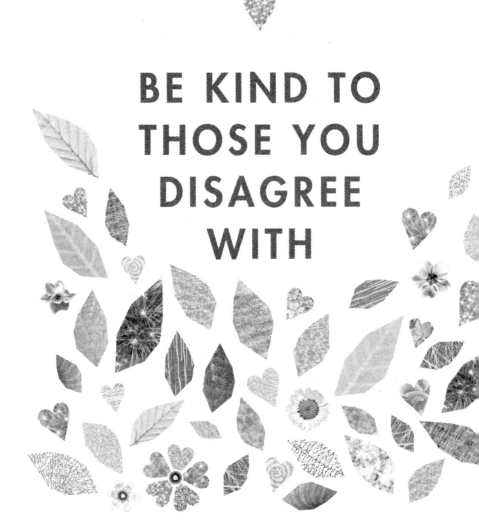

BE KIND TO THOSE YOU DISAGREE WITH

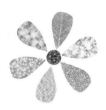

We'd all like a more peaceful world. Nobody wants news feeds filled with images of bombed cities or desperate people fleeing war zones. We know that money spent on wars would be much better spent on education, conservation, healthcare; anything but the bombs and bullets that destroy lives every day. It seems as if there has always been war, as if it is just the way of human beings, and that regretfully we have to accept it, whilst we prepare to defend ourselves.

I don't believe this has to be the way.

The peace that we crave starts with each of us. We can begin to imagine the possibility that humans can behave differently, by behaving differently ourselves. I know that this is easier said than done, when faced with someone who is irritating or offending you and what you'd really like to do is throw a custard pie in their face (or worse). But we can make a powerful start by being kinder to those we disagree with.

How does this work, day to day? What happens if you meet someone whose opinion is so offensive to you, so absolutely contrary to your beliefs and what you hold dear: what then? How do we move forward and demonstrate being peaceful under such duress? I don't believe anyone has ever changed their mind by being shouted at or called names. There are plenty of reasons to be angry. But there are also plenty of ways to progress.

We can make a powerful start
by being kinder to those
we disagree with.

As you prepare for an uncomfortable conversation with someone who doesn't agree with you, consider this: perhaps *you* are wrong. Maybe your long-held opinion should be challenged. Maybe there is something you can learn from each other. Perhaps being uncomfortable is the feeling you get when you are about to discover something life-changing. You could begin changing someone's opinion, and help them to see something from a different perspective. This has to be an improvement on the mini-war of two people shouting at each other, or the isolation of two people not listening to each other. If you're angry, have hope that things can improve, and take action by beginning the conversation.

A while ago I was creating a new theatre show with a group of young people about Utopia. One of the girls said to me: 'The trouble with Utopia is, everyone would agree with each other, and that's so boring.' We discussed whether conflict always makes for a more exciting story. She continued, 'But we don't want war either.' We talked about how new ideas and solutions could come out of disagreements, so that they can be progressive and helpful, and interesting (in the end we created a fun vision of the future which included talking animals and solar-powered cars).

Without dissent and differing opinions, the world would be a very bland place, as the young people in my theatre group discovered. Finding a way to disagree constructively and with kindness is one of the most important lessons for our times.

366 days

I was on a train with a man with a very loud posh voice.
I realised I was making assumptions about him (basically
that he wouldn't be very nice, based on no evidence except
my own bias). So I made an effort to talk to him. He turned
out to be funny, sweet and a good conversationalist. I was
pleased to be proved wrong. Notice when you make negative
assumptions about people, talk to them, allow yourself to be
surprised and challenge your prejudices – we all have them.

LISTEN

Don't shout. If you're hoping to change someone's mind,
then shouting probably won't help. Telling someone they're
wrong won't work either; it could make them defensive.
Be gentle, kind and neutral, and you're more likely to have
a more productive and interesting conversation. They are
much more likely to listen if you have shown some respect
for their opinion.

Make sure you are actively listening, not just being quiet
until they have stopped and it's your turn to talk again. Be

aware if you are just waiting for an opportunity to disagree with what's been said. If you don't listen fully, you may miss something that you can learn from. Don't assume that the speaker has nothing important or valuable to say; you don't know that.

Try:

- Turning to face the speaker so they have your full attention and can see that.

- Not to interrupt.

- Letting them know that you understand that this is a strong belief or opinion for them.

- To keep an open mind.

- To think the best of them whilst you are listening. It will help you to keep an open mind.

Ask questions:

- To clarify anything you weren't sure about, so there is less room for misunderstandings.

- To help you understand how they came to these opinions.

CHALLENGE
AND BE CHALLENGED

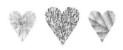

If someone says or does something that you believe to be wrong, then it is possible to challenge it with kindness. Tell them what they did, and then direct them towards useful information ('there's an interesting article/show/documentary I think you'd like'). If they ask you a question you don't know the answer to: find out. Arm yourself with knowledge.

Being kind does not mean passively tolerating bad behaviour, but it does give us more effective ways of challenging it. If someone challenges you, listen. Consider what they said and try to see it from their point of view. It is hard to accept you are wrong, but we all are sometimes, and admitting it takes real strength.

FIND COMMON GROUND

Try to find common ground with the person you disagree with; is there any aspect of what they are saying that rings true to you? Or sounds familiar? If so, tell them.

Be kind by acknowledging their hurt and anger if they have expressed that.

If they are hurt or angry think about situations that made you feel the same, share that information with them.

IF AN ARGUMENT HAPPENS

If an argument starts, as they sometimes do, be the first to say sorry, even if it doesn't feel like it was your fault. Be the peacemaker.

If you can, return to the part that started the row and find out what sparked it.

It might be here where things start to get really interesting, and both parties can learn a lot.

SAY THANKS

Acknowledge and thank them for the courage it took to disagree. Acknowledge your own courage in disagreeing.

KNOW WHEN TO WALK AWAY

It's OK to agree to disagree. It's OK to simply say, 'I don't share your views but thanks for sharing them.'

STICK UP FOR PEOPLE

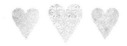

If you see someone being harassed, don't stand by; stand up for them. Keep yourself safe.

- Speak to the person who is being harassed rather than challenging the harasser.

- Ask them if they're OK and start a conversation. Focus on them, not the harasser.

- Move them away as quickly as possible.

- Report the harassment as soon as you can (only give specific information about the victim if you have their permission).

- If you're aware that in your neighbourhood a specific group of people are being harassed, look after those who might be victims, say hello, ask how they are and be friendly.

QUICK-FIRE WAYS TO SUPPORT PEACE IN THE WORLD

Begin a list of organisations, groups and people who support peace, either by being great at debating or actively campaigning for peace. Sign up to their newsletters and share stories about the peacemakers in the world.

♥ Educate yourself – there is so much for us to learn about each other. Our methods of communications have brought us closer together and this is both a gift and a challenge. The more we know and understand about each other, the less chance of conflict. Find out about other cultures by talking, reading and listening.

♥ Support charities working for peace – with donations, volunteering or fundraising.

♥ Sign petitions and share information to support people who suffer from human-rights abuses or as a result of war.

♥ Act for peace yourself. If you're angry, use it. Look for the hope, and use your energy to take positive action.

CHAPTER 7

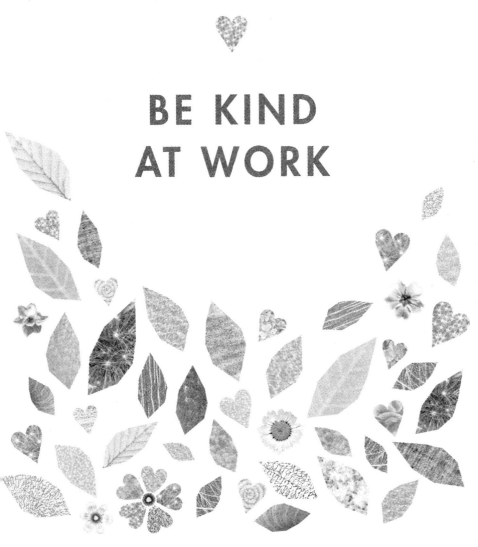

BE KIND
AT WORK

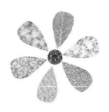

*A*s we all seem to be working longer and longer hours, it is more important than ever to be kind at work. We have to enjoy our time outside work, of course, but work is part of life, so it deserves as much attention as anything else. We may as well try to make our working lives happier for ourselves and those around us, and with all those hours spent with colleagues and co-workers, work provides perhaps our biggest opportunity to be kind.

Kindness in words creates confidence.

Kindness in thinking creates profoundness.

Kindness in giving creates love.

LAO TZU

My best boss ever was Sarah. Sarah began a tradition in our small office of serving tea and homemade cakes at 4 p.m., so everyone could get together and away from their desks for a short while. She used a mixture of charm and gentle persuasion to get everyone to join in, and it made for a much jollier working atmosphere. Her cakes were delicious, too. She once ran after me as I left work to give me a Christmas present. Everyone who worked with her was happier for doing so.

366 days

Inspired by Sarah, later I tried a few acts of kindness in the workplace myself, including: leaving treats/notes on people's desks, making people cups of tea/coffee/strange herbal infusions, getting everyone to sign birthday cards for each other, taking homemade cakes in for everyone.

Now I work on my own most of the time (not because of the strange herbal infusions, I hope . . .), but all the things I have learned about being kind at work still apply. I've broken them down over the next few pages.

IN PERSON

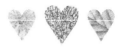

Don't underestimate the power of a nice smile. Or if you can't smile, then glower with a certain enigmatic allure. Seriously, smiling goes a long way towards improving someone's day, as does simply remembering to say hello and goodbye to everyone you work with, asking how they are, getting to know and remember your co-workers' names. Do these things every day and other people will follow your example.

If you have to deliver a message to someone, at least once a day get up and deliver it in person instead of by email. Stretch your legs.

MIND YOUR MANNERS

It's all too easy to be unintentionally rude or brusque when you are stressed and busy. We can imagine it takes more time to be polite, but you'll find that people will help you out more if they feel appreciated. So remember to say thank you. Say 'well done' whenever you notice someone has done a good job and pay attention to your co-workers' efforts. Return calls and emails promptly; don't make someone's job harder or make them feel unimportant by not responding. Be brief, but do reply asap. Always work as hard as anyone working with or for you, try your best to be on time, and assume that everyone else is working hard and doing their best, even if you don't know what their work is.

> Give someone a thank-you card if they've gone out of their way to help you or worked extra hard.

TIME FOR TEA

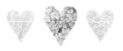

However grand your job title is, make tea. Bring in treats for everyone occasionally. You could even try making a tea chart with everyone's names and beverage specifications! If people take a break with you, take the opportunity to find out what your co-workers like to do, which films and books and hobbies they enjoy, what makes them laugh. Be aware that sometimes people just need to work without interruption. Be sensitive to this: make them a cuppa and let them get on with it.

LUNCH BREAK

Take someone for lunch who is having a hard time – if it seems appropriate enquire about it, otherwise simply have a pleasant break with them. Take the opportunity to get to know them – ask for their opinion about work matters and listen. If they're having work problems or being bullied, support them and encourage them to report it. If they tell you they feel their hard work gets overlooked, make sure people know by telling them. Sometimes it's easier to air grievances away from the workplace.

> Be nice to the new person. Introduce yourself and introduce them to others. Ask them to lunch, find out a bit about them. It can be difficult being new.

BE THE BEST BOSS

If you're in charge, lead by example: find out what would make the workplace happier and gather kindness ideas from your colleagues by creating a suggestions box. Make it so that people can pop notes in anonymously if they want – pin some of your own ideas above it to get things started. Here are some examples:

- A colouring/graffiti wall for doodling
- A charity bake sale
- Healthy snacks for everyone's desk or workplace
- Parties for everyone and their families
- A 'joke of the day' message board (even cheesy ones are fun – you could write an example)

Start a birthday calendar on the next page of all your co-workers' birthdays (with notes about whether they like to be made a fuss of or whether they prefer to keep it quiet; what kind of cake they'd like, if any, etc.). Create a copy and stick it in a place where everyone will see it.

Name	Date	Notes

BE KIND TO YOURSELF
AT WORK

Decorate your work area if possible; make yourself as comfortable and relaxed as you can be there. Get creative with your space. Acknowledge to yourself when you've done something well, and ask for feedback from someone you trust, who will be both honest and supportive of your work. Remember to take a breather. Once you've finished a task, take a moment to reflect on how it went and just relax for a few moments. Keep healthy snacks within arm's reach and don't forget to drink water and keep yourself hydrated. Do yourself a favour by getting organised – tidy your workplace and keep your calendar up to date. This will reduce stress and make your day easier.

Find time to walk outside if you work indoors, and get moving. Try these with a colleague:

- Use the stairs instead of the lift.

- Walk around the workplace as much as possible.

- Fit exercise into your working day if you can — try a class at a nearby gym at lunchtime.

- Explore what is around the area where you work — you might be near a beautiful park or an interesting gallery. Take the opportunity to find out.

Partner with a colleague and arrange to go for a walk or run one day a week.

TIME TO CHANGE?

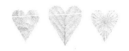

If your work is making you unhappy, carefully consider why. Is it possible for things to change and, if so, do you need help making those changes? Begin plans to change your circumstances — you may not be able to implement these immediately but you will feel better if you begin to devise a plan of action. Reward yourself for your hard work by doing something fun or relaxing.

> Reflect on your working day every day by remembering three positive things that happened. This may help you to realise that your day wasn't as bad as it seemed.

BOSSY BOOTS

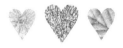

If you are your own boss, be the sort of boss that you would like to work for. Decide on your hours and stick to them. Give yourself breaks at regular times. Establish a routine – one that works for you. Enjoy the advantages of being in charge of your own hours and relish those freedoms. Get out. Take breaks – go for a walk in the park or a potter round the local shops. Make connections with other people who work alone too, in the same field as you – it's a great way of building a support network and sharing information.

Meet someone for coffee – even for just half an hour – so that each day you connect with someone face to face.

Redefine success – your own way. You won't get a prize for working the most hours in a week or making the most money. Ask yourself what your idea of a good life is. If the answer is getting by on the money from your part-time job and spending your spare time in the countryside with a metal detector seeking ancient coins with your dog, and that is what you are already doing, you have succeeded. But be kind on your way too: a good measure of success is how much happiness you've brought into people's lives, and how much you've made the world a better place, by being kind.

Redefine success

— your own way.

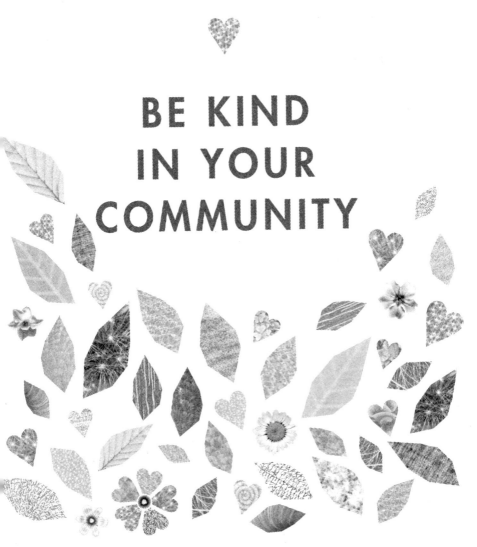

CHAPTER 8

BE KIND IN YOUR COMMUNITY

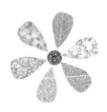

*M*any of us now live in cities and towns that are changing very rapidly. Shiny new glass tower blocks spring up like mushrooms, seemingly overnight. Suddenly, we find we have a lot more neighbours, and I wonder how many of us know each other? Connecting with your neighbours and wider community can make your home seem safer and friendlier, plus, on a practical level, if you're friends with the family next door you have someone to take in parcels/feed the cat when you're on holiday, so it's a win-win situation.

I am fortunate enough to live along the route of the London Marathon. Hundreds of people line the streets to cheer on the incredible efforts of the runners as they stream past. Every year on my street, we enjoy a great, inspiring day (not everyone can say that Mo Farah and a man dressed as a T-Rex ran past their house as they were eating breakfast. It's impossible not to have a smile on your face at this sight). Gradually our marathon-day celebrations have got more extravagant. Now, every year, I put a shout-out on social media and we make banners to hang in the window for anyone running, local kids bake and sell cakes to raise extra money for good causes, people dance, chat and laugh with each other. It is London at its absolute best. Even if you don't have a big public event like this that gets everyone out on the streets, there are loads of things you can do to spread kindness in your community.

366 days

I took my new neighbours a 'welcome to our street' card with some ice creams for their kids. I wasn't sure to begin with whether they were pleased or not, but a few months later, they tidied up my garden whilst I was away after overhearing me say I hadn't time to do it. Now we exchange gifts from time to time, and have door-step catch-ups whenever we see each other.

BE A GOOD NEIGHBOUR

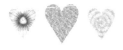

Say hello and stop for a chat whenever you get the opportunity. If you've made a birthday cake and have some left over, offer it to your neighbours instead of throwing it away. Offer to help with shopping, babysitting, dog-walking, etc. Let them know they can ask if they need to. Ask for help yourself too – people are usually happy to be helpful and they'll feel more able to ask you if they need something.

> Be considerate: let your neighbours know if you might be noisy (if you're having a party just invite them!).

PARTY!

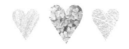

Small
Invite your neighbours round for a cup of tea – get to know them better.

Medium
If you've space, have a get-together with a few of your neighbours – give everyone the chance to meet each other.

Large
If you're feeling energetic, throw a big one! Find a community space (church hall, scout hut, etc.) and ask everyone to bring something to eat or drink if they are able – if it works you could make it a regular event.

Mega
You could even revive the good old-fashioned street party – if you can deal with the traffic!

NEWCOMERS

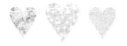

If you've noticed that someone new has moved in, this is a great opportunity for kindness. Send them a card to welcome them to the neighbourhood (you could even make one if you're feeling crafty). Compile a list for them of the top ten things to do/places to go in your area – or you could hand-draw a map. Make some notes on the next page of the top ten things near you: it's a great way of focusing on the positives in your area (if you come up with more than ten, all the better!). Deliver your new neighbour a 'starter' kit – a box or basket with a few essential items that everyone needs when they first move in: tea, biscuits, fruit juice, etc.

Top Ten

....

....

....

....

....

....

....

....

....

....

USE SOCIAL MEDIA

Start a community Facebook group, Instagram or Twitter account for your local park or street. Use them as digital noticeboards. Share information about the best places to get breakfast, coffee and locally sourced produce, suggest the best pubs and cafes, support new local businesses by mentioning them, support neighbours' projects and connect like-minded people with each other. Keep it positive: use to it to help people feel pride in their community.

> Post stuff that you don't need any more online, but which a neighbour might find useful – encourage others to do the same and reduce fly-tipping!

LOCAL VOLUNTEER OPPORTUNITIES

Volunteering can mean you get to know people locally who share your interests, learn new skills, and feel good about yourself for helping out. There are usually loads of local organisations that could do with a hand. You could:

- Help animals.
  (try www.bluecross.org.uk/volunteer-pets)

- Help the homeless.
  (try www.crisis.org.uk/pages/volunteer.html)

- Help deliver food to people in need.
  (try www.royalvoluntaryservice.org.uk/volunteer)

- Help wildlife and the environment.
  (try www.wildlifetrusts.org/volunteer)

- Help young people.
  (try www.barnardos.org.uk/get_involved/volunteering/volunteering_with_children_and_young_people.htm)

SHOP LOCALLY

Visit independent shops and markets – speak to and get to know the people who work there (instead of being admonished by a disembodied voice who tells you there's an 'unexpected item in the bagging area'). If you support the local economy it will benefit your community – you will help unique local shops to thrive, create local jobs and keep your area interesting and lively.

Window boxes

Make your place beautiful – plant window boxes, or a few bulbs if you have a front garden or patio. It's a kindness to passers-by and your neighbours to give them something gorgeous to look at.

'SOMEONE SHOULD DO SOMETHING ABOUT THAT . . .'

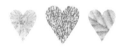

Be that someone!

- Too much rubbish everywhere? Pick up litter as you walk (take gloves and a spare bag with you) or have a ten-minute tidy of the park once a week.

- Worried about the welfare of homeless people in your neighbourhood? Find out what resources are available locally to help them. Speak with them. Take them a care kit: socks, a flask and a travel card or bus pass are great, as well as toiletries.

- Be a 'guerrilla gardener' and plant a few bulbs in that scruffy patch of earth you pass every day.

- Find out about community gardening schemes; officially adopt a patch of land and transform it.

QUICK-FIRE, FUN WAYS TO BE KIND IN THE COMMUNITY

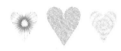

- Have a clear-out and leave a box labelled 'free stuff' outside your home. Take what's left to a local charity shop.

- When you take items to your local charity shop, as an extra bit of fun why not leave notes inside coat pockets or inside bags or book pages? Imagine how brilliant it would be to find a note saying, 'Hello, I hope you like this bag/coat/book – I loved it.'

- It's usually very cheap to put a card up in your local newsagent's. Use it to make a fun joke or to advertise a little piece of happiness or wisdom. This idea is inspired by a newsagent's window near where I live. I noticed that some of the signs in the window were daft and hilarious ('Darts trophy for sale. Would be suitable for someone called Dave Carter. £5 ONO.') I've copied this idea and done a few of my own.

- The park keeper, the postie, the firefighters, the doctors, the pharmacists, the woman who always has time to chat in the local shop: write them a thank-you card or note. These people make your community work, and sometimes their jobs aren't the most glamorous!

- Fundraising for a good cause as a community is a great way of bringing people together – you could fundraise for a community garden, or for a day trip out for the local sheltered housing. Make it fun – you could organise a film night, garden party or auction.

- These days there are loads of community libraries and food banks run by hardworking volunteers who need your help! First, drop by and check that new books would be welcome and if there are any in particular they need. Ask people to drop off books to you and then deliver them.

- Do the same with cans and dry food for your local food bank (again, check what they especially need), or toys for your local playgroup.

CHAPTER 9

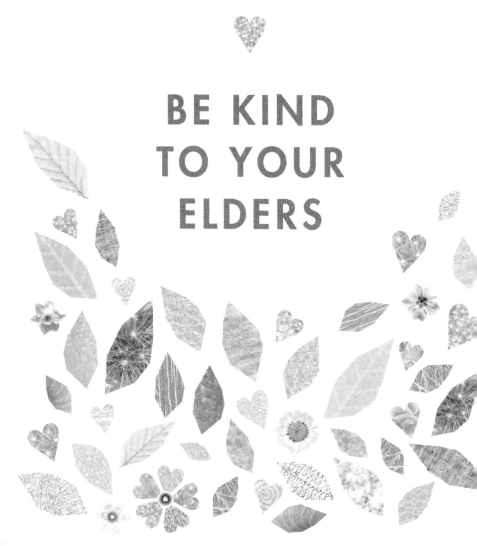

BE KIND
TO YOUR
ELDERS

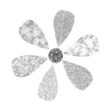

Life expectancy in some parts of the world has hugely increased – many of us are now living well into our 80s, 90s and beyond. The time is right to improve attitudes towards the elderly – to ensure that later life can be as happy and fulfilling as possible.

A huge challenge to many older people is loneliness. Children leave home, friends, relatives and partners might pass away, people finish work and may drift away from contact with their friends and colleagues, poor health or reduced mobility can mean that some people aren't out and about as much as they used to be.

The organisation Campaign to End Loneliness has conducted detailed research into effect this has on seniors' well being, and it's shown that loneliness and social isolation are harmful to health. Lacking social connections is a comparable risk factor for early death to smoking 15 cigarettes a day, and is worse for us than obesity and physical inactivity.

As my ninety-four-year-old friend Eve said: 'Everyone gets to be young. It's only us lucky ones that get to be old.'

Eve told me she felt lucky because she lived with friends, had regular contact with her family, and had 'loads of fun' – and she's not alone. I've participated in lots of creative projects with older people, so I have witnessed the best of what later life has to offer. I have seen tea dances filled with seniors jiving the afternoon away, art exhibitions by those who have discovered a flair for painting or sculpture, plays written and performed by seniors, raucous choirs and ukulele orchestras filled with dapper gents and glamour girls in their sixties and upwards singing and playing their hearts out. For most people these years are free from work and childcare, so they can be liberating and fun. There are lots of groups available for older people to get involved in, but they're not yet available everywhere and there isn't the capacity to include everyone who might benefit. But there is plenty we can do.

The time is right
to improve attitudes
towards the elderly.

366 days

A few months into my year of acts of kindness, I saw a gentleman on the bus wearing a very stylish hat. I told him so and we got talking. His name was Alvin. He told me he hadn't spoken to anyone for a couple of days and was glad to chat. After that I made a focused effort to connect with elders more. There are some ideas over the next few pages that could apply to your older relatives, elderly neighbours or those you pass in the street. By the way, I still see Alvin and we have since become good friends. He has become a positive influence on my hat choices.

A little thought and a little kindness
are often worth more than
a great deal of money.

OUT AND ABOUT

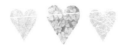

Say hello: make a point of smiling and saying hello to seniors as you are going about your day. Don't underestimate this simple action – if someone greets you, you no longer feel invisible and you may begin to think maybe the outside world is pretty friendly after all.

Get talking: when you live alone it's very easy not to speak with anyone from day to day. A good place to strike up a conversation is if you see a senior walking their dog. Ask about the pet and you'll soon be chatting away. If you find yourself next to an older person, just ask, 'How are you?' If you think an older person may have trouble hearing or has memory problems, make sure to speak clearly without shouting. Go slowly; be patient.

Offer your seat: if you are able. Make a habit of looking around you to notice those with mobility issues. Many people do not have the confidence to ask.

IN THE NEIGHBOURHOOD

- Introduce yourself to your elderly neighbours; get to know their names.

- Find out when their birthdays are and drop a card in — many older people don't get any or many birthday cards.

- Check in with them at least once a week just to see how they are.

- Ask them how long they've lived in the neighbourhood; discover local stories.

- Ask after their health so you can be aware of any assistance they may need.

- Check to see if they need help with pets. Take an older person's dog for a walk or offer to clean the cat's litter box.

- Ask if they need any other help with shopping, housework, posting letters, picking up prescriptions and medicines, etc.

STAYING IN/GOING OUT

- Spend time with older people, find out what they like to do and help them do it, and find something you can enjoy doing together.

- Invite them over for a chat and a cup of tea. Just spend time hanging out.

- Surprise an elderly neighbour with a home-cooked meal – take something round or invite them to dinner.

- Arrange a night out they'd like – to the pub, cafe or theatre. It is surprising how infrequently some people get out of their own homes, and how quickly going out can become nerve-wracking.

VOLUNTEER

- Pop into your local sheltered housing office and see if they need any practical help – or you could offer to put on a game of bingo, a party or a quiz.

- Volunteer for an organisation that supports older people, such as Age UK. They run 'befriending services' and are always on the lookout for more people to help. Check out what is going on locally here: www.ageuk.org.uk

LEARN TO LISTEN

- If you have older relatives, make time to visit or phone and ask how they are.

- Take the opportunity to get to know them as people, not just as 'Mum and Dad'. Discover the stories you don't know by asking questions – find out who Mum's first love was, what Dad wanted to be as a child, what Granddad thinks is better about the world now.

- Look at photos together; make a scrapbook of words and images, or a video or podcast of their memories and life story. Make them feel special.

Conduct a fun interview with an older relative or friend, with entertaining questions like 'Who would you invite to your dream dinner party?' etc. Type up the interview and give it to them.

A CHANGING WORLD

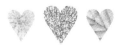

The world is changing so rapidly now that many older people feel left behind, and as if their experiences and knowledge are worth little, their opinions not of interest.

♥ Ask them to share their thoughts and opinions about the world.

♥ Find out if they need help with the internet or with their phone/TV/iPad.

♥ Ask them if there is anything they'd like to learn and help. Do a skill swap – I can guarantee there will be things to learn from them, too.

♥ Ask their advice about changing careers, getting married or starting a family. Lots of things don't change – we still fall in love, get our hearts broken, try to work out what to do with our lives, and strive for happiness. Remember, they've been there before. They can help.

SHARING STORIES

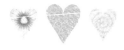

My friend Clara, seventy-nine, once surprised me by teaching me how to make a mojito, and regaling me with tales of the wild dances of her youth. Old folk are as complex and interesting as all other humans, of course, with as wide a variety of opinions, experiences and outlooks as younger people have, so be prepared to be surprised and have some prejudices challenged. Most of us know the basics from our history lessons: the dates when wars began and ended, the names of presidents and queens and the lives of 'great men and women'. But history is more than the facts, and you have an opportunity every time you speak with a senior to learn something incredible, surprising and inspiring about the past. Listening is one of the kindest things we can do for each other.

CHAPTER 10

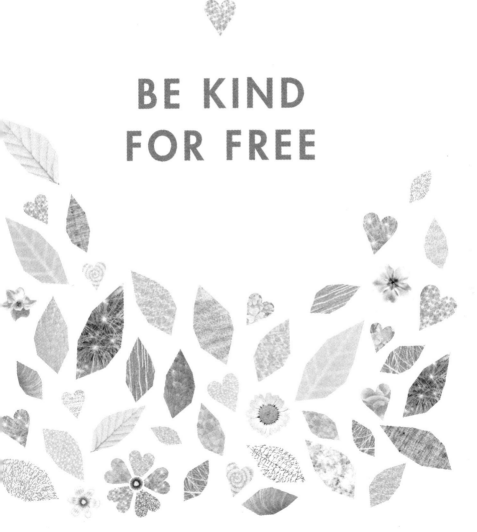

BE KIND
FOR FREE

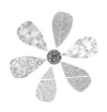

That old saying 'the best things in life are free' still holds true. Laughing until your stomach aches, listening to the birds sing, having a good chat with an old friend, watching the sunset or sunrise, seeing a rainbow, dancing, jumping in puddles on a rainy day, kicking through the autumn leaves, having a lie-in, playing air guitar whilst listening to rock classics, spending time with people who make you happy, noticing the spring flowers popping up: all of that is soul food and good to remember.

I admit to spending lots of money in my 'kindness mission' in the beginning (I'm a long way from being rich, but even if I was, I'm not convinced spending money is always the best way of being kind anyway). I did a lot of buying presents and giving money away – I don't regret it for one moment but it wasn't sustainable. To avoid bankruptcy and also because my mum kept telling me off for it, I set about devising more imaginative and creative ways to be kind for free – there are so many fun ways to do it. It means you can always be kind, in good times and bad, and helps you realize the most generous acts of kindness often involve giving your time, attention, focus and love, rather than cash.

By the end of the first year I had given so much away it made me realize how little we need really, how much our possessions can weigh us down by taking up our time and space, as we have to take care of them, store them, organise and clean them. I am a natural hoarder so for me to make this discovery was a real triumph!

The most generous acts of kindness often involve giving your time, attention, focus and love, rather than cash.

366 days

I find books incredibly hard to part with, but I had run out of shelf space and was in imminent danger of being buried under a paperback avalanche. I discovered some fun and creative ways to part with them: I started leaving books in cafes, at bus stops, on train seats, at the dentists, with sticky notes on the cover saying 'I'm free, please take me' and a hand-written message inside. Other books I posted out to friends, some I boxed up and took to our local community library. Some I handed to perfect strangers whilst I was out and about. I've kept this up since, and recommend passing on books once you have read them, it makes every one you buy for yourself a gift for someone or somewhere else, eventually.

Kindness clutter

Getting rid of all your unwanted belongings is a free, fun and fabulous way to be kind. You'll have more space in your home, and there are lots of different ways of doing this. Ask yourself how much you want or need something – if your answer is less than say, 7/10, give it away to someone who will love it more.

A recipe for kindness

Cooking and sharing food is a great way of being kind to yourself and others. Have a dinner party – but ask all your guests to bring a home-cooked dish. Work out beforehand who would prefer to make sweet or savoury dishes, so you don't end up with seven trifles and no main courses! This way nobody should have to spend any more than they usually would for their own dinner, and no one has to work too hard. Ask each guest to bring their recipe, and after the dinner party you could compile a 'cook book' of your special night, to share with all your guests. Maybe you could even turn this into a monthly event, at someone else's place each time?

Table service

Often when people are very busy or isolated they don't have time to prepare proper meals. You could visit and deliver a pre-cooked meal! Have some fun with this and make them a menu card, and next to the food place a candle and a flower on a tray. Be prepared for them not to answer the door – have the food covered in readiness for this, leave it on the doorstep, ring the bell and run away like a magic delivery service. (I know this means foxes might eat it. Take that chance.)

Free gifts

Homemade gifts are the greatest. Have a think about what you could gift someone for free. If you are a champion in the kitchen – get cooking. Could you paint a picture, knit a hat, or write a poem? If you've got green fingers you could give a gift of a plant you have grown or some seeds for someone to grow their own. If you play an instrument or sing you could serenade someone. If you're handy you could make something. Discover or rediscover your creative side and make something for someone.

Magical mystery tour

If you have the time and someone asks you for directions, why not take them there yourself? If you're lucky enough to live somewhere that gets a lot of visitors, this is such a delight – you get to meet people and feel proud of the amazing place you live. Feeling lost or bewildered in an unfamiliar place and having a friendly face to help you is one of those 'restore your faith in humanity' moments. I know, I have been helped many times as I have the sense of direction of a drunken rocking horse, so I often have to ask for help, even with GPS.

The currency of kindness

If you know someone who is mega busy, find out what you can do for them. Offer your time and help with washing up, housework, shopping, helping them to get organised, etc. Some people find it incredibly difficult to ask for help – so surprise them with a helping hand.

Be silly,
be honest,
be kind.

RALPH WALDO EMERSON

QUICK-FIRE KINDNESS

- Give blood. This could save someone's life in an emergency or help those who need long-term treatments.

- Join the NHS organ donor register and help someone to live when you die.

- Get back in contact with someone you've lost touch with – it's one of the great joys of social media.

- Think about skills you could share – like helping someone with a CV, or teach them to ride a bike or swim, computer skills or gardening.

- Give a massage.

- Let someone who is sleep deprived have a lie-in. Do the morning chores whilst they snooze.

- Tell someone a story – there are few greater pleasures than being read to. If you're able – make a story up. Or find one of your favourites and retell it.

- Play games. Take time to play with the children in your life, and encourage the adults in your life to play too. Arrange a card night, or a football/rounders match in the park.

- ♥ Write someone a letter. It's such a rare delight to receive something in the post that isn't a bill; it's guaranteed to put a smile on someone's face.

- ♥ Go for a walk with a loved one. Find somewhere beautiful. Take your time.

- ♥ Waste time with someone. Just hang out, make no plans, do what takes your fancy.

- ♥ Listen. Talk. Ask someone how they are and give them your undivided attention, paying no attention to the clock.

LAST BUT NOT LEAST . . .

Do not underestimate kindness. It's not weakness; it can take great strength. It includes learning to forgive and love yourself and others; it requires enough courage to be open and to think the best of yourself and others. It takes guts to see and to seek the best in humans, but it can also be a lot of fun and it can fill your life with a real kind of magic, and it allows you to see the possibility that the world can work differently. It is a quiet kind of revolution.

In the end, if you consciously practise daily kindness it will become automatic, just like breathing. It will transform your life and connect you more deeply to everything. Try it. Join us. Let's show everyone that kindness can change the world.

FURTHER READING

Some useful and inspiring resources:

ONLINE

www.sundayassembly.com a non-religious congregation

www.actionforhappiness.org promoting happiness globally

www.positive.news a constructive journalism magazine

www.theschooloflife.com educational organisation concerned
with living wisely and well

craftivist-collective.com using craft to engage people in social
justice

www.campaigntoendloneliness.org tackling the threat of
loneliness

www.ageuk.org.uk supporting older people

www.kindnessuk.com charity promoting kindness

peopleunited.org.uk charity exploring how art can promote
kindness

balance.media magazine focusing on well-being and kindness

www.meatfreemondays.com vegetarian ideas and recipes from
the McCartneys

www.rspb.org.uk for guidance on what to feed wild birds and
when

BOOKS

Why Kindness is Good For You by David Hamilton PhD
Self Compassion by Kirsten Neff PhD
How to Change the World by John-Paul Flintoff

ACKNOWLEDGEMENTS

Thanks to the many people who advised, helped and encouraged me over the years, including: Gareth Brierley, Jackie Russell, Natalie Russell, Kimberley Trim and their families; Lola Fandango, Christine Entwisle, Asif Iqbal, Cindy Townsend, Steve Richards, Kirsty McQuire, Kirsty Harris, Dan Thompson, Mark Williamson, Reverend Pete Sainsbury, Jack Trow, Tom Andrews, Darin Jewell, Sophie Scott, Jamie Glassman, Billy Bragg, Jess Worrall, Sadie Cook, Fred De Faye, Annie Calverley, Siobhain Furlong, Sarah Tully, J. P. Flintoff, Sarah Corbett, Stella Duffy, Lucy Anne Holmes, Ross Mullan, Kate Baily, Jules Craig, Vera Chok, Vanessa Woolf-Hoyle, Penny Pepper, Paul McVeigh, Gaylene Gould, Eve Yarker, Keith Williams, Sharon Calcutt Cheadle, Jenni Morris, Denise The Lady Flower, Stewart Who?, Gerald Kyd, Sam Scott Wood, Krishna News and the Patel family, Keith Williams, Gill Lloyd and Arts Admin, Tessa Walker and Birmingham Rep, Ade Berry and Jacksons Lane, Raidene Carter and The Albany, Meet Me At and Deptford Lounge, Matthew Couper and Deptford X, Helen Medland, Tim Harrison and The Basement, Colin D. Anthony and the staff of London Underground, Radio 4 *Saturday Live*, Usborne Books, Graham Robson, Susan Kelly, and all at Ivy Kids/Quarto, Sunday Assembly, Zoe Charles and The Cheek of It!, all at Southbank Centre, Penny Dreadful Theatre Company, Olivia Morris and all at Orion, and the people of Deptford.

Lastly, the boy at the post office whose name I don't know, who accepted a bit of change from me and changed my life forever.

ABOUT THE AUTHOR

Bernadette Russell is an author and storyteller who lives and works in Deptford, south-east London. She is co-director of the arts organisation White Rabbit, with Gareth Brierley. She has created shows for organisations including the National Theatre, the Southbank Centre and Birmingham Rep. Her children's books are published by Ivy Press. She was selected as one of the Southbank Centre's 'Change Makers' in 2015 for her project *366 Days of Kindness*, which was the inspiration for this book. She is a columnist for *Balance* magazine, has been a speaker for Action for Happiness and Sunday Assembly, and gives talks on kindness and compassion for schools and organisations here and in the USA.

www.366daysofkindness.com
— where you can read Bernadette's diary of kindness

www.bernadetterussell.com
— where you can read about all of her work

Twitter @betterussell
Facebook @bernadetterussellwrites
Instagram @bernadetterussell